Ketogenic Diet Cookbook

The Essential Guide for Beginners

Rosa Hall

Furthermore, the transmission, duplication or reproduction of any of the following work including specific information will be considered an illegal act irrespective of if it is done electronically or in print. This extends to creating a secondary or tertiary copy of the work or a recorded copy and is only allowed with express written consent from the Publisher. All additional rights reserved.

The information in the following pages is broadly considered to be a truthful and accurate account of facts and as such any inattention, use or misuse of the information in question by the reader will render any resulting actions solely under their purview. There are no scenarios in which the publisher or the original author of this work can be in any fashion deemed liable for any hardship or damages that may befall them after undertaking information described herein.

Additionally, the information in the following pages is intended only for informational purposes and should thus be thought of as universal. As befitting its nature, it is presented without assurance regarding its prolonged validity or interim quality. Trademarks that are mentioned are done without written consent and can in no way be considered an endorsement from the trademark holder.

TABLE OF CONTENTS

Introduction: Getting Acquainted with the Ketogenic Diet

The fact that you purchased this cookbook is proof that you are someone who is very much interested in changing their life. Because the Ketogenic Diet isn't some temporary fix, it's a health improvement for the long haul. Here in this chapter we will explain exactly what Ketogenic is, *what it isn't*, the benefits derived of Ketogenic, Ketogenic foods, and how to start your very own ketogenic meal plan.

Ketogenic Explained

A ketogenic diet is carried out with the express purpose of placing the body into the metabolic state of "ketosis". When the body reaches a state of ketosis, it begins to burn fat as a primary fuel source rather than glucose from carbohydrates. You see, for most of us, normally our body is running off of all the bread, pasta, and other grains we eat—this is the primary fuel source, while all fat is stored away and stockpiled for later use. This is fine when you are young, skinny, and your fat stores are low.

But as we get older and continue this grain heavy, carb loaded diet, our fat stores begin to grow in the form of stubborn belly fat, flabby arms, and the like. In order to get rid of them, the Ketogenic Diet focuses on shifting the diet away from carb heavy grains, and toward consuming higher levels of fat and protein. Yes, that's right. In order to get rid of some fat, *you have to eat some fat*! If may seem like an oxymoron—contradiction of the highest level, but it is the truth.

Because it is only when you start eating fatter foods, that the body begins to get used to the idea of fat being burned as the primary fuel source. A body lacking carbs but being infused with fat, simply has no choice but to switch gears and begin burning fat as its main source of energy. It's like the body is a diesel engine realizing it's been fed gas for far too long, and suddenly switches itself back to diesel! As the body switches to burning up fat for fuel, all of those stubborn fat deposits are drained, and burned up! To sum it all up—by reprogramming the body's metabolic state, to burn fat instead of storing it—you can lose a whole lot of weight!

Benefits from Ketogenic

Being able to rapidly burn up fat is an easy to understand benefit of a ketogenic diet, but fat burn is not the only way in which one can benefit from ketogenic. Ketogenic can improve a wide variety of mechanisms in the body. Helping to facilitate better circulation, improved metabolism, and even more efficient cognitive function. The ways in which one can reap the reward of ketogenic are numerous indeed. Here is just a brief sampling of the positive attributes that have been ascribed to a dedicated regimen of the ketogenic diet.

- Improved Cognitive Function
  Yes. It is true. A regular ketogenic regimen can improve cognitive function. This has been borne out in studies dating all the way back to 500 BC! You see, even the ancients were accustomed to

fine tuning their diets in a ketogenic manner. And by the time of the early 20th Century it was discovered that ketogenic could even treat something as devastating as epileptic seizures. It is the reinforcement of vital neurons in the body that ketogenic facilitates, that allows this reversal of epileptic symptoms to occur. Another benefit of this improved cognition is an increased capacity of memory, which has been cited as a possible treatment for age reality deficiencies such as "Alzheimer's" as well. Improved cognitive function can indeed be gained from a ketogenic diet.

- Canceling Out Cancer

Cancer has been a dread illness for centuries, and successful cures and treatments have been few and far between. But as bad as it is—there are promising new studies that have demonstrated the ability of a ketogenic diet to slow down and even reset the metabolic rate of cancer itself! Results are still pending, but if ketogenic can indeed cancel out cancer, it would certainly be a true game changer for us all.

- Elimination of Cardiovascular Disease

  Ketogenic has been able to reduce the onset of cardiovascular illness considerably simply by better stabilizing metabolic rates, and normalizing the pressure of the body's blood. Regular ketogenic helps to bring triglycerides and "HDL" down to more manageable levels, helping to negate, and even reverse clogging of the arteries

- Reduction in Inflammatory Illness

  Inflammation has been cited as a cause of many disorders in recent years—affecting people with everything from arthritis to irritable bowel syndrome. Many things in the environment and our diet can contribute to inflammation; ketogenic however, is able to significantly reduce the body's inflammatory response, thereby getting at the root cause of many kinds of chronic illness. Ketogenic reduces calories and thereby reduces damaging free radicals, allowing the body to heal itself of all kinds of inflammation.

- Feeling More Energized

  One of the most immediate benefits that most ketogenic dieters experience, is a feeling of being more energized. It's usually in the middle of the first week of the diet that you begin to feel a natural jolt of energy. This is due to the fact that your body has managed to cleanse itself of harmful free radicals, as well as perfectly balance out blood pressure, blood sugar, and even insulin. And as soon as your body switches off of carbs, and starts running off of your stored fat deposits as fuel, you will indeed feel much more energized than usual!

- More Efficient Urinary System

  When the urinary system is out of whack, with important organs such as the kidneys, and bladder not functioning properly—you could be in for a really rough ride when it comes to your health. And afflictions of gout, kidney stones, and outright kidney failure, might not be too far behind. Ketogenic however, is able to reboot this important system of the body, clear out calcified kidney stone deposits, prevent gout, and ensure that your entire urinary system runs smoothly for the long haul.

- Reduction in Acid Reflux

In our society of overly processed foods, incidents of acid reflux have become more and more common, and now it's very well near epidemic. If you take the time to think about it, you will find that either yourself or someone you know has chronic bouts of acid reflux. And this same acid reflux has become more and more severe. With some cases so bad that the sufferer's throat and even their mechanism to swallow properly have been irrevocably damaged. Stomach acid you see, is a very powerful agent designed to dissolve solid food, but when it rises up out of the stomach and into the esophagus, that same acid just might burn a hole in your throat! The ketogenic diet however is able to combat these problems and stop acid reflux in its tracks, bringing the naturally occurring chemistry of the mouth, throat, and stomach back to a normal, and healthy state.

- Improved Vision

If your vision has been affecting you as of late, you just might want to see what a ketogenic diet can do for you. You see, a strict ketogenic regimen is fully capable of reducing blood sugar, and it is elevated blood sugar that often—quite literally—blurs our vision. This is why so many suffer from diabetic blindness, all due to dangerously elevated blood sugar. Ketogenic will bring these blood sugar levels back down to normal however and will improve your vision as a result.

- Decreasing the Incidence of Diabetes

  Probably one of the things that ketogenic is best known for, is its ability to battle diabetes. Being diabetic is one of the major scourges of our time, with those who suffer from the illness literally losing life and limb during the course of the disease. But ketogenic since it is able to reboot the body's entire metabolic process, and better regulate hormones such as insulin—ketogenic can, and will indeed decrease the incidence of diabetes.

12

Ketogenic Foods

- Fish
- Poultry
- Beef
- Eggs
- Non-Starchy Vegetables
- Natural Fat
- Cheese
- Olive Oil
- Almond Oil
- Coconut Oil
- Avocados
- Coffee
- Nuts
- Butter

Non-Ketogenic Foods

- Many Fruits
- Potatoes
- Pasta
- Rice
- Bread
- Milk
- Soda
- Legumes (beans, chickpeas, and peanuts)
- Wheat flour
- Millet
- Sorghum

Starting Your Meal Plan

As you start the ketogenic diet you should create for yourself a clear meal plan. This should consist of a hearty breakfast that is full of fat (yes fat) so that you can start your day with plenty of energy, and remain full in between eating windows. You can then skip lunch altogether and opt for either fasting the rest of the day or eating a very light dinner. Alternately you could also choose to skip breakfast and lunch both, and then begin the next eating window at dinnertime, with a hearty and healthy meal at the end of the day, in addition to perhaps a good dessert!

However, you start your meal plan just make sure you stick to it, and you will come out on top!If it helps you to do so, you should consider keeping a food journal, and writing down everything you eat. You can also plot out on the calendar every meal for the following week in advance. Some have even utilized AI assistants such as Amazon's Alexa to help keep them on track. Ketogenic works well within a finite structure, so once you set up your meal plan be sure to adhere to it. With ketogenic it pays to be organized, and at least some small level of meal planning can be tremendously beneficial.

Chapter 1: Breakfast with Ketogenic

More often than not, how we start our day is going to have a major role in how it is that we finish our day. If we wake up hungry, and with a severe lack of energy, and don't do anything to stave off those hunger pains, and help improve our stamina, we are going to end our day just as lackluster as we had started it. On the other hand, if we start up our day with all the nutrients we need, and an adequate energy supply to boot, we will have a much greater chance of taking the day by storm. Here in this chapter you will find a full listing of all the recipes you will need to kick off your day in style!

Almond Flour Pancakes

It's truly amazing what a little bit of almond flour can do—this delicious recipe tastes as great as it will make you feel!

Prep Time: 4 min and 30 seconds

Passive Time: 0 min

Cook Time: 24 min

Total: 28 min and 30 seconds

Serves: 1-2

Ingredients:

- 3 eggs
- ½ cup of almond flour
- ¼ cup of cream cheese
- 1 tsp of butter
- ½ tsp of cinnamon

Directions:

1. Add your 3 eggs, your cup of almond flour, your ¼ cup of cream cheese, your ½ tsp of cinnamon to a blender and hit the blend button.

2. After blending the ingredients for 30 seconds, unplug blender and set to the side.

3. Now place a large frying pan onto a burner set for high heat and deposit your tsp of butter inside.

4. Now pour half of your almond flour mixture out of the blender and into the pan, and cook each side for about 6 minutes, before transferring cooked pancake to a plate.

5. Repeat the process again with the other half.

6. Serve when ready.

Nutritional Information:

Calories: 150

Total Fat: 14 g

Saturated Fat:3g

Cholesterol: 61 mg

Total Carbs: 4 g

Sugar: 1 g

Fiber: 0 g

Sodium: 232 mg

Protein: 6 g

Broccoli Breakfast Muffins

Ok I know what some of you may be thinking—*Broccoli for breakfast?* But I can assure you, this blend of Broccoli and whole wheat flour is absolutely delicious! These Broccoli Breakfast Muffins more than pass the taste test!

Prep Time: 5 min

Passive Time: 15 seconds

Cook Time: 25 min

Total: 30 min and 15 seconds

Serves: 3-4

Ingredients:

- 2 tsp of ghee
- 1 cup of chopped broccoli
- 2 cups of almond flour
- 2 eggs
- 1 cup of almond milk

- 2 tablespoons of nutritional yeast

- 1 tsp of baking powder

- ½ tsp of sea salt

Directions:

1. Get started by preheating your oven to 375 degrees, and greasing a muffin tin with your 2 tsp of ghee.

2. Set the tin to the side, and while the oven heats up, take out a medium sized mixing bowl and add your cup of chopped broccoli, your 2 cups of almond flour, your 2 eggs, your cup of almond milk, your 2 tablespoons of nutritional yeast, your tsp of baking powder and your ½ tsp of sea salt.

3. Stir all of these ingredients together well, before evenly pouring the mixture into each of the cups of your muffin tin.

4. Now place the muffin tin into the oven and allow it to cook for about 25 minutes.

5. Turn off your oven, allow to cool for about 15 seconds, and then serve whenever you are ready.

Nutritional Information:

Calories: 101

Total Fat: 4 g

Saturated Fat: 1g

Cholesterol: 3 mg

Total Carbs: 12 g

Sugar: 0.5 g

Fiber: 1 g

Sodium: 270 mg

Protein: 4 g

Ketogenic Waffles

Everybody likes waffles right? And with this ketogenic friendly variety you don't have to worry about wrecking your whole diet! Ketogenic Waffles—you've just got to try it!

Prep Time: 5 min

Passive Time: 30 seconds

Cook Time: 3 min

Total: 8 min and 30 seconds

Serves: 5-6

Ingredients:

- 5 eggs
- 6 ounces of cream cheese
- ¼ cup of soy protein powder
- 1 tsp of baking powder
- 1 cup of whole almond flour

- 1 tablespoon of whey protein powder

- 1 tsp of heavy cream

Directions:

1. Add your 5 eggs, your 6 ounces of cream cheese, your ¼ cup of soy protein powder, and your tsp of baking powder to a blender, hit the blend button, and thoroughly blend together for about 30 seconds.

2. Once blended, pour ingredients into a waffle iron, shut the iron, and bake for about 3 minutes.

3. Take waffles out of iron, and place them on a plate.

4. Serve with whatever ketogenic based toppings you like.

Nutritional Information:

Calories: 317

Total Fat: 30 g

Saturated Fat: 16g

Cholesterol: 277 mg

Total Carbs: 2 g

Sugar: 0.5 g

Fiber: 0.5 g

Sodium: 357 mg

Protein: 8 g

Eggs and Chile Pepper Breakfast

Eggs, chili peppers, tomato and cheese! For one spicy breakfast—try this one out for size!

Prep Time: 5 min

Passive Time: 0 min

Cook Time: 14 min

Total: 19 min

Serves: 7-8

Ingredients:

- 1 cup of chopped green chili peppers
- 1 cup of sour cream
- 1 tablespoon of grated parmesan cheese
- 1 cup of grated cheddar cheese
- 1 cup of chopped tomato
- ½ tsp of salt
- 1 tsp of pepper
- 14 eggs

Directions:

1. Set your oven to 350 degrees.

2. While your oven is heating up, get out a glass baking dish and add your cup of chopped green chili peppers, your cup of sour cream, and your tablespoon of grated parmesan cheese to the pan.

3. Now crack your 14 eggs into the pan, and season with your ½ tsp of salt, and your tsp of pepper.

4. Place your pan of ingredients into the oven and allow to cook for about 10 minutes.

5. After your 10 minutes have passed, take the dish out of the oven, and sprinkle your cup of grated cheddar cheese over the ingredients.

6. Place back into the oven and cook for an additional 4 minutes.

7. Once your 4 minutes have passed, take the dish out of the oven and sprinkle top with your cup of chopped tomatoes.

8. Serve when ready.

Nutritional Information:

Calories: 311

Total Fat: 15 g

Saturated Fat: 0g

Cholesterol: 425 mg

Total Carbs: 6 g

Sugar: 2 g

Fiber: 2 g

Sodium: 390 mg

Protein: 14 g

Beefy Avocado Bowl

Beef and Avocado in a bowl provides you what you need to get going!

Prep Time: 5 min

Passive Time: 0 min

Cook Time: 5 min and 30 seconds

Total: 10 min and 30 seconds

Serves: 2-3

Ingredients:

- 2 cups of diced onion
- 1 pound of ground beef
- 2 cups of diced mushroom
- ½ tsp of pepper
- ½ tsp of salt
- 1 tsp of paprika
- 1 tablespoon of olive oil
- ¼ cup of chopped avocado

- 1 tablespoon of chopped black olives

- 2 eggs

Directions:

1. Place a frying pan onto a burner set for medium- high heat, and add your tablespoon of olive oil to the pan.

2. Now add your 2 cups of diced onion, followed by your 2 cups of diced mushrooms, and your ½ tsp of salt.

3. Mix and stir well as the ingredients cook over the next 3 minutes.

4. Next, deposit your pound of ground beef into the pan, followed by your tsp of paprika, stir and cook for another 2 minutes.

5. Now add your 2 eggs to the pan and stir them into the ingredients as well, cooking for about 1 more minute.

6. Finally, add your ¼ cup of chopped avocado, and your tablespoon of chopped black olives.

7. Stir and cook for another 30 seconds before serving.

Nutritional Information:

Calories: 616

Total Fat: 38 g

Saturated Fat: 6g

Cholesterol: 407 mg

Total Carbs: 26

Sugar: 5 g

Fiber: 8 g

Sodium: 1008 mg

Protein: 51 g

Blueberry and Granola Bowl

Here's yet another breakfast in a bowl! It doesn't leave too much to the imagination, but if you need a simplistic breakfast that will fill you up right, look no further than this blend of Blueberry and Granola!

Prep Time: 5 min

Passive Time: 0 min

Cook Time: 0 min

Total: 5 min

Serves: 1-2

Ingredients:

- ¼ cup of chopped blueberries

- 1 tablespoon of chopped dark chocolate

- 1 tablespoon of chopped pecans

- 1 tablespoon of lemon juice

Directions:

1. Deposit your tablespoon of lemon juice, followed by your ¼ cup of chopped blueberries, your tablespoon of chopped dark chocolate, and your tablespoon of chopped pecans.

2. Simply stir these ingredients together and your Blueberry and Granola bowl is finished!

Nutritional Information:

Calories: 205

Total Fat: 3 g

Saturated Fat: 1g

Cholesterol: 9 mg

Total Carbs: 29 g

Sugar: 20 g

Fiber: 4 g

Sodium: 77 mg

Protein: 3 g

Ham and Cheese Omelet

It's the cheesiest omelet you will ever find anywhere!

Prep Time: 5 min
Passive Time: 0 min
Cook Time: 5 min
Total: 10 min

Serves: 1-2

Ingredients:

- 1 tablespoon of butter
- 1 tablespoon of olive oil
- ¼ cup of shredded cheddar cheese
- ¼ cup of chopped ham
- 1 tsp of sea salt
- 1 tsp of pepper
- 2 eggs

Directions:

1. Place a medium sized frying pan onto a burner set for high heat and add your tablespoon of olive oil to the pan.

2. Now add your 2 eggs into the pan, and stir them into the oil as they cook over the next 2 minutes.

3. Next, add your ¼ cup of chopped ham, followed by your ¼ cup of shredded cheddar cheese, your tsp of sea salt, and your tsp of pepper.

4. Stir everything together well as the ingredients cook for another 3 minutes.

5. Finally, turn burner off, allow about 30 seconds to cool and solidify, and serve when ready.

Nutritional Information:

Calories: 250

Total Fat: 9 g

Saturated Fat: 3g

Cholesterol: 205 mg

Total Carbs: 19 g

Sugar: 4 g

Fiber: 1 g

Sodium: 289 mg

Protein: 14 g

Bacon-Cheddar Biscuit in a Cup

Yes, you heard right! Here you will find juicy bacon, creamy cheese, and filling biscuit, all in one convenient cup!

Prep Time: 1 min
Passive Time: 0 min
Cook Time: 55 seconds
Total: 1 min and 55 seconds

Serves: 1

Ingredients:
- 1 egg
- 2 tablespoons of butter
- 3 tablespoons of almond flour
- ½ tsp of baking powder
- ¼ cup of crumbled (cooked) bacon
- 1 tablespoon of shredded cheddar cheese

- 1 tablespoon of shredded white cheddar
- 1 tablespoon of chopped chive
- 1 tsp of salt
- 1 tsp of Mrs. Dash

Directions:

1. Deposit your egg, your 2 tablespoons of butter, your 3 tablespoons of almond flour, your ½ tsp of baking powder, your ¼ cup of crumbled bacon, your tablespoon of shredded cheddar cheese, your tablespoon of shredded white cheddar, your tablespoon of chopped chive, your tsp of salt, and your tsp of Mrs. Dash.

2. Stir the ingredients together and place in your microwave.

3. Cook for about 55 seconds.

4. Take out and flip upside down over a bowl or plate.

5. This Bacon-Cheddar Biscuit in a Cup is ready to eat!

41

Nutritional Information:

Calories: 170

Total Fat: 8 g

Saturated Fat: 1g

Cholesterol: 5 mg

Total Carbs: 19 g

Sugar: 9 g

Fiber: 2 g

Sodium: 509 mg

Protein: 9 g

Chapter 2: Lunchtime Ketogenic

Lunch is a time to recharge your depleted batteries. Having that said, you need something that is filling, and satisfying, as well as being perfectly Ketogenic based! Here in this chapter you will find several great Lunchtime Ketogenic recipes.

Ketogenic Hamburgers

Would you like a burger for lunch? Well—that's no problem at all with these Ketogenic Hamburgers!

Prep Time: 5 min
Passive Time: 0 min
Cook Time: 10 min

Total: 15 min

Serves: 2-3

Ingredients:

- 1 pound of ground beef
- 1 tsp of salt
- ½ tsp of pepper
- 1 tsp of oregano
- 2 tablespoons of diced tomato
- 2 tablespoons of shredded cheddar
- 4 lettuce leaves

Directions:

1. Deposit your pound of ground beef, your tsp of salt, your ½ tsp of pepper, and your tsp of oregano, into a large bowl.
2. Now use your hands to shape these ingredients into two distinct hamburger patties, and place them into a frying pan.

3. Set the burner on high, and cook each side of the patty for about 5 minutes.

4. Once cooked, arrange 2 leaves on two separate plates.

5. Place a cooked patty on a lettuce leaf, top each one with a tablespoon of shredded cheddar, followed by a tablespoon of diced tomato, and then top with the remaining lettuce leaf.

6. Your Ketogenic Hamburgers are ready to serve!

Nutritional Information:

Calories: 485

Total Fat: 24 g

Saturated Fat: 12g

Cholesterol: 124 mg

Total Carbs: 15 g

Sugar: 5 g

Fiber: 4 g

Sodium: 1420 mg

Protein: 21 g

Afternoon Chicken Wings

There isn't anything that can quite compare to an afternoon of stuffing your face with chicken wings! And unlike those binges at BW3's back in college—these chicken wings won't make you feel guilty later on!

Prep Time: 7 min
Passive Time: 1 min
Cook Time: 45 min
Total: 53 min

Serves: 4-5

Ingredients:
- 20 chicken wings
- 1 cup of grated parmesan cheese
- 1 tsp of chopped parsley
- 1 tsp of garlic powder
- 1 tsp of white pepper

- 1 cup of melted butter

Directions:

1. First, go through your chicken wings, rinsing them off and patting them dry with napkins, or paper towels, and set them to the side.

2. Next, set your oven to 375 degrees, get out a baking dish, and slightly grease it, placing it to the side as well.

3. Now deposit your cup of grated parmesan cheese, your tsp of chopped parsley, your tsp of garlic powder, your tsp of white pepper, and your cup of melted butter into a medium sized mixing bowl.

4. Stir these ingredients together well.

5. Take each of your chicken wings and dip them into the mixture, before arranging them inside of your greased baking dish.

6. Place dish into the oven and cook for about 45 minutes.

7. Take out, allow 1 minute to cool, and serve.

Nutritional Information:

Calories: 285

Total Fat: 19 g

Saturated Fat: 5g

Cholesterol: 120 mg

Total Carbs: 3 g

Sugar: 4 g

Fiber: 1 g

Sodium: 289 mg

Protein: 22 g

Sweet and Sour Chicken

Here is another chicken recipe classic! You're going to love this one!

Prep Time: 4 min
Passive Time: 0 min
Cook Time: 12 min
Total: 16 min

Serves: 3-4

Ingredients:

- 4 boneless, skinless chicken breast halves
- 2 tablespoons of coconut oil
- 1 tsp of black pepper
- 2 tablespoons of butter
- 1 tablespoon of chopped onion
- ½ cup of diced tomatoes
- 1 cup of chicken broth

- 1 cup of white wine

- 1 tsp of hickory smoke liquid

- 1 tsp of garlic powder

- 1 tablespoon of sugar

Directions:

1. Set your oven to 350 degrees, get out a casserole baking dish, and grease it with one of your tablespoons of coconut oil, and place it to the side.

2. Now place a small saucepan onto a burner set for medium-high heat and add your 2 tablespoons of butter, followed by your tablespoon of chopped onion, your ½ cup of diced tomatoes, your cup of chicken broth, your cup of white wine, your tsp of hickory smoke liquid, your tsp of garlic powder, and your tablespoon of sugar, and cook for about 8 minutes.

3. Next, take your boneless, skinless chicken breasts and cut them up into small pieces.

4. Place a large frying pan onto a burner set for high heat add your remaining tablespoon of coconut oil, before depositing your chicken into the pan.

5. Stir and cook the chicken for about 4 minutes.

6. Season the cooked chicken with your tsp of black pepper, before moving them to the greased casserole dish.

7. Pour your small saucepan of ingredients over the chicken in the dish, and place the casserole dish into the oven.

8. Cook for about 45 minutes.

9. Serve up your chicken while it's hot and juicy!

Nutritional Information:

Calories: 411

Total Fat: 9 g

Saturated Fat: 1g

Cholesterol: 47 mg

Total Carbs: 7 g

Sugar: 7 g

Fiber: 2.5 g

Sodium: 232 mg

Protein: 35 g

Tuna Crunch Lunch

If you would like a lunch with some fish and crunch, try this Tuna Crunch Lunch!

Prep Time: 5 min
Passive Time: 0 min
Cook Time: 5 min
Total: 10 min

Serves: 2-3

Ingredients:
- 1 can of tuna
- ½ cup of chopped onions
- 2 tablespoons of chopped parsley
- ½ tsp of salt
- ¼ tsp of dried thyme
- 1 tsp of black pepper
- 1 tablespoon of chopped pecan
- 1 tablespoon of coconut oil

- 2 eggs

Directions:

1. Open up a can of tuna and drain it of any water inside, before depositing the tuna into a mixing bowl.

2. Now add your ½ cup of chopped onions, your 2 tablespoons of chopped parsley, your ½ tsp of salt, your ¼ tsp of dried thyme, your tsp of black pepper, your tablespoon of chopped pecans, and 2 eggs to the bowl and stir everything together well.

3. Place a large frying pan onto a burner set for high heat, and add your tablespoon of coconut oil.

4. Pour your tuna/egg mixture into the pan, and cook for about 5 minutes.

5. Serve when ready.

Nutritional Information:

Calories: 298

Total Fat: 23 g

Saturated Fat: 1g

Cholesterol: 247 mg

Total Carbs: 2 g

Sugar: 1 g

Fiber: 2 g

Sodium: 886 mg

Protein: 21 g

Salty Scampi

A little salt and a lot of scampi can go a long way!

Prep Time: 5 min
Passive Time: 0 min
Cook Time: 10 min
Total: 15 min

Serves: 2-3

Ingredients:

- ½ cup of olive oil
- 1 tablespoon of lemon juice
- ½ cup of white wine
- 1 pound of shrimp
- 5 tablespoons of butter
- 1 tsp of garlic powder
- 1 tsp of salt
- 1 tsp of pepper

Directions:

1. Set your oven for 275 degrees.

2. While your oven is heating up, place a large frying pan onto a burner set for medium heat.

3. Now add your ½ cup of olive oil, your tablespoon of lemon juice, your ½ cup of white wine, and your 5 tablespoons of butter to the pan.

4. Stir and cook the ingredients for about 5 minutes, before adding your pound of shrimp.

5. Next, add your tsp of garlic powder, your tsp of salt, and your tsp of pepper.

6. Stir the ingredients together well and cook for another 5 minutes.

7. Your Salty Scampi is ready to go!

Nutritional Information:

Calories: 246

Total Fat: 11 g

Saturated Fat: 5g

Cholesterol: 230 mg

Total Carbs: 7 g

Sugar: 5 g

Fiber: 2 g

Sodium: 335 mg

Protein: 27 g

Spicy Mayo Tuna Stack

Spice, mayo and tuna stacked to perfection! All the makings of a great lunch!

Prep Time: 7 min

Passive Time: 0 min

Cook Time: 0 min

Total: 7 min

Serves: 1-2

Ingredients:

- 1 tsp of hot sauce
- 2 tablespoons of mayonnaise
- ¼ cup of mayonnaise
- 1 tsp of sea salt
- 1 tsp of black pepper
- 1 cup of guacamole
- 1 cup of chopped lettuce
- 1 can of tuna

- ½ cup of diced hard-boiled eggs

Directions:

1. First, take your tsp of hot sauce, and your 2 tablespoons of mayonnaise and deposit them into a small bowl, stirring them together well.

2. Next, take out a medium sized mixing bowl and add your ½ cup of diced hard-boiled eggs, followed by your mayonnaise/hot sauce mixture, your tsp of sea salt, and your tsp of black pepper, stir all of these ingredients together well.

3. Now get out 2 plates and create a circle with a ½ cup of your guacamole on both plates/

4. Next stack ½ of your chopped lettuce on top of the guacamole, followed by placing ½ of the can of tuna on each mound of lettuce.

5. Add your egg mixture on top of the tuna, evenly distributing it between the two plates.

6. Serve when ready.

Nutritional Information:

Calories: 219

Total Fat: 19 g

Saturated Fat: 7g

Cholesterol: 109 mg

Total Carbs: 1 g

Sugar: 4 g

Fiber: 2 g

Sodium: 224 mg

Protein: 9 g

Buffalo Chicken Strips

As you can see, if you like chicken—you are going to love ketogenic! Here is yet another great chicken-based recipe for your lunch!

Prep Time: 5 min

Passive Time: 0 min

Cook Time: 25 min

Total: 30 min

Serves: 1-2

Ingredients:
- 5 chicken breasts
- 1 cup of almond flour
- ½ cup of hot sauce
- 1 tablespoon of olive oil
- 3 tablespoons of butter
- 3 tablespoons of blue cheese crumbles
- 1 tablespoon of paprika

- 1 tablespoon of chili powder

- 1 tsp salt

- 2 tsp of pepper

- 1 tsp of garlic powder

- 1 tsp of onion powder

- 2 eggs

Directions:

1. Set the temperature of your oven to 420 degrees.

2. While your oven is warming up, go ahead and get out your ramekin, and add your tablespoon of paprika, your tablespoon of chili powder, your tsp of salt, your 2 tsp of pepper, and your tsp of onion powder, stirring these ingredients together well.

3. Now spread out your chicken breasts onto a cooking sheet and cut them in half.

4. Sprinkle about half of your ramekin mixture onto your chicken breasts, before flipping them over and adding the remain half to the other side of your chicken as well.

5. Now place your cooking sheet into the oven and cook for about 25 minutes.

6. Serve when ready.

Nutritional Information:

Calories: 342

Total Fat: 19 g

Saturated Fat: 3g

Cholesterol: 60 mg

Total Carbs: 24 g

Sugar: 15 g

Fiber: 2 g

Sodium: 220 mg

Protein: 29 g

Bacon, Chicken, and Sausage Stir Fry

This dish is so good it took three animals to make it! Bacon, Chicken, and Sausage Stir Fry!

Prep Time: 5 min
Passive Time: 0 min
Cook Time: 13 min
Total: 18 min

Serves: 2-3

Ingredients:

- 4 bacon, cheddar, and chicken sausages
- 3 cups of chopped broccoli
- 3 cups of chopped spinach
- ½ cup of parmesan cheese
- ½ cup of tomato sauce
- ¼ cup of red wine
- 1 cup of water
- 2 tablespoons of salted butter

- 2 tsp of chopped garlic

- ½ tsp of red pepper flakes

Directions:

1. Take your 4 bacon, cheddar, and chicken sausages and slice them into neat, uniform slices.

2. Place a medium saucepan onto a burner set for high heat and add your cup of water to the pan, before adding your bacon, cheddar, and chicken sausage slices.

3. Now add your 3 cups of chopped broccoli to the pan and cook the ingredients for about 5 minutes, periodically stirring the ingredients around in the pan.

4. Next, add your 2 tablespoons of butter, followed by your 2 tsp of chopped garlic, continue to stir and cook for 3 more minutes.

5. Finally add your ½ cup of tomato sauce, your ¼ cup of red wine, and your ½ tsp of red pepper flakes, stirring the ingredients together well, and cooking for another 5 minutes.'

6. Serve whenever you are ready to do so.

Nutritional Information:

Calories: 311

Total Fat: 10 g

Saturated Fat: 2g

Cholesterol: 34 mg

Total Carbs: 5 g

Sugar: 3 g

Fiber: 1.5 g

Sodium: 342 mg

Protein: 6 g

Chapter 3: Dinnertime Ketogenic

At the end of the day you are going to need something that is nourishing and replenishing for your spent bodily batteries. Here in this chapter we provide you with some of the best recipes to make as you get ready to conclude another great ketogenic day. Have Dinnertime with Ketogenic!

Ketogenic Turkey Casserole

This one is filling and satisfying. Turkey, scallions, celery, cheese, and more—It has everything that you need to succeed!

Prep Time: 7 min
Passive Time: 0 min

Cook Time: 20 min

Total: 27 min

Serves: 4-5

Ingredients:

- 2 cups of diced (cooked) turkey chunks
- 2 cups of diced celery
- 5 tablespoons of chopped scallions
- 1 cup of basic mayonnaise
- 1 tablespoon of lemon juice
- 1 tablespoon of olive oil
- ½ cup of chopped almonds
- 1 cup of grated cheddar cheese
- ½ cup of crushed pork rinds

Directions:

1. Deposit your 2 cups of diced turkey chunks, your 2 cups of diced celery, your 5 tablespoons of chopped scallions, your

cup of basic mayonnaise, and your tablespoon of lemon juice, and stir together well.

2. Now get out an additional small bowl and add your ½ cup of chopped almonds, your cup of grated cheddar cheese, and your ½ cup of crushed pork rinds, and set to the side for a moment.

3. Set your oven's temperature for 355 degrees, get out a casserole baking dish and grease the dish with your tablespoon of olive oil.

4. Now place your turkey mixture of ingredients into the dish and layer your pork rind mixture on top.

5. Place into the oven and cook for about 20 minutes.

6. Serve when ready.

Nutritional Information:

Calories: 301

Total Fat: 9 g

Saturated Fat: 5g

Cholesterol: 70 mg

Total Carbs: 27 g

Sugar: 2 g

Fiber: 1 g

Sodium: 209 mg

Protein: 24 g

Beef Stroganoff

Just check out this hearty helping of Beef Stroganoff! This is a real classic and a great recipe for both those on and off of the ketogenic diet.

Prep Time: 3 min

Passive Time: 0 min

Cook Time: 9 min

Total: 12 min

Serves: 3-4

Ingredients:

- 1 pound of beef tenderloin
- 1 tsp of salt
- 1 tsp of pepper
- 1 cup of chopped mushrooms
- 1 tablespoon of coconut oil
- 1 tsp of butter

- 1 cup of beef broth

- 1 cup of sour cream

- 2 tablespoons of chopped parsley

Directions:

1. Place your pound of beef tenderloin onto a clean cutting board and slice it into long, thin strips, and lay out onto a large plate or platter.

2. Now place a medium sized frying pan onto a burner set for high heat, and add your tablespoon of coconut oil, followed by your beef tenderloin strips.

3. Cook your meat evenly for about 2 minutes on each side, before adding your cup of chopped mushrooms and cooking for another 5 minutes.

4. Next, add your cup of beef broth, followed by your cup of sour cream, and top with your 2 tablespoons of chopped parsley.

5. Serve when ready!

Nutritional Information:

Calories: 379

Total Fat: 9 g

Saturated Fat: 5g

Cholesterol: 61 mg

Total Carbs: 31 g

Sugar: 2 g

Fiber: 2 g

Sodium: 354 mg

Protein: 22 g

Baked Fish and Zucchini

Fish and Zucchini baked to perfection! Just as nutritious as it is delicious! Bit right in!

Prep Time: 5 min

Passive Time: 0 min

Cook Time: 15 min

Total: 20 min

Serves: 4-5

Ingredients:

- 4 skinned whitefish fillets
- 1 tsp of salt
- 1 tsp of black pepper
- 1 tablespoon of butter
- 1 cup of grated Parmesan cheese
- ¼ cup of chopped zucchini
- 1 tablespoon of chopped parsley
- 1 tablespoon of olive oil

Directions:

1. Set your oven's temperature for 380 degrees.

2. While your oven is heating up, deposit your 4 skinned white fish to the baking dish, and season with your tsp of salt, tsp of black pepper and half of your cup of grated cheese.

3. Now deposit your ¼ cup of chopped zucchini over the mixture and place the baking dish into the oven.

4. Cook for about 10 minutes before taking out and drizzling your tablespoon of olive oil, and tablespoon of chopped parsley over the top of the ingredients.

5. Return the dish to the oven and cook for another 5 minutes.

Nutritional Information:

Calories: 417

Total Fat: 35 g

Saturated Fat: 18g

Cholesterol: 186 mg

Total Carbs: 23 g

Sugar: 7 g

Fiber: 2 g

Sodium: 201 mg

Protein: 4 g

Ketogenic Chicken Pot Pie

Remember that classic pot pie you loved when you were a kid? Well—here's the completely ketogenic version of it! This is a ketogenic rendition of a comfort food classic that will make you look forward to dinner!

Prep Time: 10 min
Passive Time: 25 min
Cook Time: 20 min and 45 seconds
Total: 55 min and 45 seconds

Serves: 2-4

Ingredients:

- 2 tablespoons of butter
- 2 cups of chopped chicken
- 1 tsp of salt
- 1 tsp of black pepper
- 1 cup of chopped celery

- ½ cup of diced onion

- 1 cup of chopped cauliflower

- ½ cup of chicken broth

- ½ cup of heavy cream

- 1 cup of shredded mozzarella

- 2 tablespoons of cream cheese

- ½ cup of hemp hearts

- ¼ cup of coconut flour

- ½ tsp of herbes de provence

- ¼ tsp of poultry seasoning

- 2 eggs

Directions:

1. Deposit your 2 cups of chopped chicken, followed by your tsp of salt, and your tsp of black pepper, into a medium sized mixing bowl, and place to the side for a moment.

2. Now add your 2 tablespoons of butter to a medium sized frying pan and place it onto a burner set for high heat.

3. Add your cup of chopped celery, your ½ cup of diced onion, your cup of chopped cauliflower to the pan and cook for about 5 minutes.

4. Next, add your chicken mixture to the pan, stir and cook for an additional 5 more minutes.

5. Go back to your chicken mixture and scoop it into 4 individual pie pans, and put to the side for now.

6. Now get out a heat resistant bowl and add your cup of shredded mozzarella cheese, and place in your microwave, melting the cheese for about 45 seconds.

7. Take out the melted cheese and stir it together until it is of one nice and smooth consistency.

8. Next, add in your ½ cup of hemp hearts, your ¼ cup of coconut flour, your tsp of herbes de provence, your ¼ tsp of poultry seasoning, and your 2 eggs, and thoroughly stir the ingredients together.

9. After this, take your (clean) hands and knead the dough together well, and allow to stand for about 25 minutes.

10. Once 25 minutes have passed, shape the dough into 4 distinct balls.

11. Now use a rolling pin to flatten the balls out.

12. Place each flattened disc of dough over the meat in your pie pans

13. Now place these pie pans onto a cooking sheet and put them into your oven.

14. Set the oven's temperature for 400 degrees and cook for about 15 minutes.

15. Enjoy!

Nutritional Information:

Calories: 317

Total Fat: 22 g

Saturated Fat: 9g

Cholesterol: 57 mg

Total Carbs: 10 g

Sugar: 3 g

Fiber: 3 g

Sodium: 220 mg

Protein: 17 g

Ketogenic Fried Steak

This fried steak will make you thank the chef who made it! And if that's you—you can go ahead and give yourself a pat on the back because this dish is delicious!

Prep Time: 4 min

Passive Time: 10 min

Cook Time: 9 min

Total: 23 min

Serves: 1-2

Ingredients:

- 16-ounce rib eye steak
- 1 tsp of sea salt
- ½ tsp of black pepper
- 1 tablespoon of coconut oil
- 3 tablespoons of unsalted butter
- 1 tablespoon of chopped onion

Directions:

1. Take your steak out of the refrigerator and leave it out at room temperature for about 10 minutes.

2. While your steak is sitting out, go ahead and put a large frying pan onto a burner set for high heat.

3. Cook the steak for about 2 minutes on each side.

4. Now lower your heat down to medium, and add your 3 tablespoons of unsalted butter, your tablespoon of chopped onion, and your tablespoon of coconut oil.

5. Stir and cook the ingredients into the pan for about 5 minutes.

6. Serve when ready.

Nutritional Information:

Calories: 255

Total Fat: 9 g

Saturated Fat: 3g

Cholesterol: 114 mg

Total Carbs: 3 g

Sugar: 7 g

Fiber: 2 g

Sodium: 347 mg

Protein: 25 g

Mustard Salmon

Sink your teeth into this dish! Just put some mustard on that salmon and call it a day!

Prep Time: 5 min

Passive Time: 0 min

Cook Time: 10 min

Total: 15 min

Serves: 3-4

Ingredients:

- 16 ounces of salmon fillets
- ½ tsp of sea salt
- 1 tsp of black pepper
- ½ cup of stone ground mustard
- 2 tablespoons of MCT oil

Directions:

1. Get out a large cooking sheet and line it with parchment

2. Lay out your salmon on the parchment, spacing them evenly apart on the sheet.

3. Evenly sprinkle your ½ tsp of sea salt, and your tsp of black pepper on the fish.

4. Next, deposit your ½ cup of tone ground mustard, and 2 tablespoons of MCT oil into a small bowl and thoroughly stir together.

5. Drizzle this mixture over your fish.

6. Place your salmon into the oven and set the temperature to 420 degrees, and cook for about 10 minutes.

7. Serve up while it's nice and hot!

Nutritional Information:

Calories: 209

Total Fat: 10 g

Saturated Fat: 2g

Cholesterol: 100 mg

Total Carbs: 8 g

Sugar: 2 g

Fiber: 1 g

Sodium: 147 mg

Protein: 25 g

Chicken Piccata

Four chicken thighs seasoned with pepper, sea salt, garlic, and parsley. This chicken comes garnished with everything that you need!

Prep Time: 3 min
Passive Time: 0 min
Cook Time: 7 min
Total: 10 min

Serves: 3-4

Ingredients:

- 4 chicken thighs
- 1 tsp of black pepper
- ½ tsp of sea salt
- 2 tablespoons of butter
- 1 tablespoon of chopped garlic
- ¼ cup f chicken broth
- 3 tablespoons of lemon juice

- 2 tablespoons of capers

- 1 tablespoon of chopped parsley.

Directions:

1. Arrange your 4 chicken thighs in a large frying pan, and sprinkle your tsp of black pepper and ½ tsp of sea salt over the chicken.

2. Now set your burner on high heat and add your 2 tablespoons of butter, followed by your tablespoon of chopped garlic, your ¼ cup of chicken broth, your 3 tablespoons of lemon juice, your 2 tablespoons of capers, and stir everything together as it cooks for 7 minutes.

3. After this, top with tablespoon of chopped parsley and serve.

Nutritional Information:

Calories: 177

Total Fat: 10 g

Saturated Fat: 3g

Cholesterol: 18 mg

Total Carbs: 14 g

Sugar: 1 g

Fiber: 2 g

Sodium: 160 mg

Protein: 6 g

Cinnamon Beef Stew

Hold on tight folks, because this Cinnamon Beef Stew will knock your socks right off!

Prep Time: 10 min

Passive Time: 0 min

Cook Time: 2 hours and 51 min

Total: 3hours and 1 min

Serves: 2-3

Ingredients:

- ½ pound of ground beef
- 1 cup of beef broth
- 1 tablespoon of coconut oil
- ½ cup of chopped onion
- 1 tsp of orange zest
- 1 tablespoon of orange juice
- 1 tsp of chopped thyme
- 1 tablespoon of chopped garlic

- 1 tsp of cinnamon
- ½ tsp of soy sauce
- ½ tsp of fish sauce
- 1 tsp of rosemary
- ½ tsp of sage
- 1 bay leaf

Directions:

1. Go ahead and place a medium sized frying pan onto a burner set for high heat and add your tablespoon of coconut oil to the pan.
2. Next, add your ½ pound of ground beef, followed by your ½ tsp of salt, and your tsp of pepper.
3. Stir and cook for about 3 minutes.
4. Now add in your ½ cup of chopped onion, your tsp of orange zest, your tablespoon of chopped garlic, and your tablespoon of orange juice, stirring and

cooking the ingredients into the pan for another 2 minutes.

5. Next, add your cup of beef broth, your tsp of cinnamon, your ½ tsp of soy sauce, and your ½ tsp of fish sauce, stirring and cooking for 1 additional minute.

6. After this, transfer your ingredients to a crock pot and add your tsp of rosemary, your ½ tsp of sage, and your bay leaf on top.

7. Cook ingredients inside your crock pot for about 2 hours and 45 minutes on high.

8. Serve when ready.

Nutritional Information:

Calories: 396

Total Fat: 27 g

Saturated Fat: 2g

Cholesterol: 35 mg

Total Carbs: 7 g

Sugar: 4 g

Fiber: 1 g

Sodium: 149 mg

Protein: 39 g

Ketogenic Szechuan Chicken

This is yet another true classic! Ketogenic Szechuan Chicken!

Prep Time: 4 min

Passive Time: 0 min

Cook Time: 21 min

Total: 25 min

Serves: 3-4

Ingredients:

- 1 pound of ground chicken

- 6 cups of spinach

- ½ cup of chicken broth

- 4 tablespoons of organic tomato paste

- 3 tablespoons of coconut oil

- 2 tablespoons of chili garlic paste

- 2 tablespoons of soy sauce

- 1 tablespoon of Erythritol

- 1 tablespoon of spicy brown mustard

- 1 tsp of salt

- 1 tsp of pepper

- 1 tsp of red pepper flakes

- ½ tsp of Mrs. Dash Table blend

- 1 tsp of chopped ginger

Directions:

1. In a medium sized mixing bowl, go ahead and add your 4 tablespoons of tomato paste, your 3 tablespoons of coconut oil, your 2 tablespoons of chili garlic paste, 1 tablespoon of spicy brown mustard, and your tsp of chopped ginger to a ramekin.

2. Now put your ramekin onto the stove and set the temperature to medium heat.

3. Next, add your pound of ground chicken, followed by your tsp of salt, and your tsp

erves: 2-3

ngredients:

- ½ cup of diced bacon (cooked)
- 1 tablespoon of butter
- 2 tablespoons of chopped shallots
- 1 tsp of chopped garlic
- 1 cup of chopped mushrooms
- 1 tsp of dried thyme
- 4 ounces of brie cheese rind
- 1 cup of chicken broth
- 1 tsp of sea salt
- ½ tsp of black pepper

Directions:

1. Deposit your ½ cup of diced bacon into a large saucepan and place it onto a burner set for high heat.

of pepper, allow this to heat up for about 1 minute.

4. After 1 minute has passed go ahead and add your 6 cups of spinach, followed by your ½ tsp of Mrs. Dash table blend, and your tsp of red pepper flakes.

5. Stir and cover the pan, reducing the heat down to low.

6. Allow to simmer for about 20 more minutes.

7. After 20 minutes have passed, this Ketogenic Szechuan Chicken is ready to serve!

Nutritional Information:

Calories: 179

Total Fat: 9 g

Saturated Fat: 9 g

Cholesterol: 43 mg

Total Carbs: 10 g

Sugar: 2 g

Fiber: 2 g

Sodium: 238 mg

Protein: 15 g

Chapter 4: Salads, Sou

Not everything you are going
lunch and dinner, some things
between! And here in this
introduce to you a wide variety
and side dishes that
interchangeable. Mix and matc
would like!

Mushroom and Bacon Soup

There are no ifs, ands, or buts al
going to love this soup!

Prep Time: 5 min

Passive Time: 0 min

Cook Time: 10 min

2. After this, add your cup of chicken broth, your tablespoon of butter, followed by your 2 tablespoons of chopped shallots, and your tsp of chopped garlic.

3. Now add your cup of chopped mushrooms, and your tsp of dried thyme to the pan, and stir and cook the ingredients for about 5 minutes.

4. Next, add your 4 ounces of brie cheese rind, your tsp of sea salt, and your ½ tsp of black pepper.

5. Again stir, and cook for about 5 more minutes.

6. Serve while hot!

Nutritional Information:

Calories: 497

Total Fat: 42 g

Saturated Fat: 5g

Cholesterol: 40 mg

Total Carbs: 9 g

Sugar: 3 g

Fiber: 4 g

Sodium: 438 mg

Protein: 21 g

Ketogenic Quesco Fresco

This is a great snack for any day of the week!

Prep Time: 4 min

Passive Time: 0 min

Cook Time: 1 min and 30 seconds

Total: 5 min and 30 seconds

Serves: 3-4

Ingredients:

- 1 pound of Quesco Fresco
- 1 tablespoon of coconut oil
- ½ tablespoon of olive oil

Directions:

1. First, cut your cheese into small cubes.
2. Next, add your tablespoon of coconut oil, and your ½ tablespoon of olive oil to a medium sized frying pan and place it

onto a burner set for high heat, stirring and cooking the ingredients for about 1 minute.

3. Now add your cheese to the pan, cook for about 30 seconds, or until nice and crisp, and then flip over and cook for another 30 seconds.

4. This snack is ready to eat!

Nutritional Information:

Calories: 307

Total Fat: 25 g

Saturated Fat: 0g

Cholesterol: 15 mg

Total Carbs: 2 g

Sugar: 3 g

Fiber: 1 g

Sodium: 220 mg

Protein: 7 g

Side of Sautéed Mushrooms

If you like mushrooms, you are going to like Ketogenic!

Prep Time: 5 min

Passive Time: 0 min

Cook Time: 10 min

Total: 15 min

Serves: 2-3

Ingredients:

- 4 tablespoons of coconut oil
- 1 cup of chopped mushrooms
- 1 tablespoon of chopped garlic
- 2 tablespoons of chopped onions
- 1 tablespoon of chopped cilantro
- ¼ tsp of cayenne pepper
- ½ tsp of ground turmeric
- ½ tsp of sea salt

- 1 tsp of lime juice

Directions:

1. In a large frying pan, deposit your 4 tablespoons of coconut oil, followed by your cup of chopped mushrooms, your tablespoon of chopped garlic, your 2 tablespoons of chopped onions, your tablespoon of chopped cilantro, your ¼ tsp of cayenne pepper, your ½ tsp of ground turmeric, your ½ tsp of sea salt, and your tsp of lime juice.

2. Stir all of the ingredients together as they cook over the course of the next 10 minutes.

3. Turn off burner, and serve when you are ready to do so.

Nutritional Information:

Calories: 147

Total Fat: 10 g

Saturated Fat: 1g

Cholesterol: 0 mg

Total Carbs: 9 g

Sugar: 7 g

Fiber: 1 g

Sodium: 178 mg

Protein: 10 g

Cheddar Chorizo Meatball Snack

Just get a load of this great snack!

Prep Time: 10 min

Passive Time: 0 min

Cook Time: 30 min

Total: 40 min

Serves: 2-3

Ingredients:

- 1 pound of ground beef

- 1 chorizo sausage

- 1 cup of shredded cheddar cheese

- ½ cup of tomato sauce

- ¼ cup of crushed pork rinds

- 1 tsp of cumin

- 1 tsp of chili powder

- 1 tsp of kosher salt

- 2 eggs

Directions:

1. Set the temperature of your oven to 375 degrees.

2. Get out a medium sized mixing bowl and add your pound of ground beef, your chorizo sausage, your ¼ cup of crushed pork rinds, your tsp of cumin, your tsp of chili powder, your tsp of kosher salt, and eggs.

3. Stir together, and then take your (clean) hands, and use them to shape the mixture into individual balls.

4. Place these meatballs into a baking sheet lined with foil, and place them into the oven.

5. Allow to cook for about 30 minutes, before taking out and drizzling your ½ cup of tomato sauce over the meatballs.

6. This Cheddar Chorizo Meatball Snack is ready to go!

Nutritional Information:

Calories: 321

Total Fat: 14 g

Saturated Fat: 3g

Cholesterol: 44 mg

Total Carbs: 8 g

Sugar: 4 g

Fiber: 2 g

Sodium: 197 mg

Protein: 17 g

Side of Ketogenic Coleslaw

A side of coleslaw is good with—just about anything! Try this recipe out for yourself!

Prep Time: 4 min

Passive Time: 0 min

Cook Time: 6 min

Total: 10 min

Serves: 1-2

Ingredients:

- 3 cups of shredded cabbage
- ½ cup of diced bacon
- 1 tablespoon of macadamia nut oil
- 3 tablespoons of coconut vinegar
- 1 tsp of salt
- 1 tsp of pepper
- 3 tsp of Confectioners Swerve

Directions:

1. Add your 3 cups of shredded cabbage to a large mixing bowl and set to the side.

2. Now place a large frying pan onto a burner set to high head and add your tablespoon of macadamia nut oil, followed by your ½ cup of diced bacon.

3. Cook your bacon until it is nice and crispy, should take 5 minutes.

4. Now add your 3 tablespoons of coconut vinegar, your tsp of salt, your tsp of pepper, and your 3 tsp of Confectioners Swerve, stir and cook with the bacon for 1 more minute.

5. Pour bacon and all other ingredients in the pan over your bowl of shredded cabbage.

6. Toss the cabbage around so that the hot ingredients marinate it thoroughly.

7. Serve when ready.

Nutritional Information:

Calories: 163

Total Fat: 9 g

Saturated Fat: 3g

Cholesterol: 25 mg

Total Carbs: 5 g

Sugar: 3 g

Fiber: 1 g

Sodium: 89 mg

Protein: 4 g

Side of Greek Asparagus

The Greeks were some of the best philosophers of the ancient world—and they also knew how to make a good side of asparagus!

Prep Time: 4 min
Passive Time: 0 min
Cook Time: 4 min
Total: 4 min

Serves: 2-3

Ingredients:
- 1 pound of trimmed asparagus
- 2 tablespoons of coconut oil
- 1 tablespoon of chopped garlic
- 1 tablespoon of lemon juice
- 1 tsp of sea salt
- 1 tsp of pepper
- 1 cup of crumbled feta cheese

- 2 tablespoons of diced onion
- 1 tsp of olive oil

Directions:

1. Set your oven for 400 degrees
2. While your oven is warming up, coat a cooking sheet with your 2 tablespoons of coconut oil and arrange your pound of asparagus onto the sheet.
3. Now take your tsp of salt and tsp of pepper and use them to season your asparagus.
4. Next sprinkle your tablespoon of chopped garlic, and your tablespoon of lemon juice over the top of the ingredients.
5. Place your sheet of asparagus into the oven and allow it to cook for 4 minutes.
6. After 4 minutes have passed, take your pan out of the oven, and add your cup of crumbled feta cheese on top, followed by

your 2 tablespoons of diced onion, and your tsp of olive oil, drizzled evenly over the ingredients.

7. This side of Greek Asparagus is ready to serve!

Nutritional Information:

Calories: 262

Total Fat: 19 g

Saturated Fat: 3g

Cholesterol: 6 mg

Total Carbs: 11 g

Sugar: 2 g

Fiber: 3 g

Sodium: 245 mg

Protein: 15 g

Simply Ketogenic Salad

A simplistic blend of salad for any occasion.

Prep Time: 5 min

Passive Time: 0 min

Cook Time: 0 min

Total: 5 min

Serves: 1-2

Ingredients:

- 3 tablespoons of olive oil

- 2 cups of spinach

- 1 tablespoon of parmesan cheese

- 1 tsp of Dijon Mustard

- 1 tsp of curry powder

- 1 tablespoon of lemon zest

Directions:

1. Get out a small mixing bowl and add your 3 tablespoons of olive oil, followed by your tsp of Dijon Mustard, and your tablespoon of lemon zest, stirring the ingredients together well.

2. Now get out an additional bowl and add your 2 cups of spinach, your tablespoon of parmesan cheese, and your tsp of curry powder.

3. Add your small mixing bowl of the olive oil/mustard mixture onto the spinach ingredients, briefly toss together and serve.

Nutritional Information:

Calories: 203

Total Fat: 23 g

Saturated Fat: 1g

Cholesterol: 45 mg

Total Carbs: 2 g

Sugar: 6 g

Fiber: 2 g

Sodium: 138 mg

Protein: 9 g

Ketogenic Clam Chowder

The best chowder this side of Boston! You're going to love it!

Prep Time: 5 min

Passive Time: 0 min

Cook Time: 9 min

Total: 14 min

Serves: 3-4

Ingredients:

- 1 tablespoon of olive oil

- ¼ cup of diced shallots

- 1 tablespoon of Thai red curry paste

- 1 cup of chicken broth

- 1 cup of coconut milk

- 12 ounces of canned clams

- 1 tsp of sea salt

- 1 tablespoon of chopped cilantro

- ¼ cup of chopped onions
- 1 tablespoon of lime juice

Directions:

1. Deposit your tablespoon of olive oil, followed by your ¼ cup of diced shallots, into a large saucepan, and set the burner for medium-high heat, cooking the ingredients for about 1 minute.

2. After cooked for about 1 minute, go ahead and add in your tablespoon of Thai red curry paste, your cup of chicken broth, and the can of coconut milk, stirring the ingredients together as they cook another 3 minutes.

3. Next, add your 12 ounces of canned clams, your tsp of sea salt your tablespoon of chopped cilantro, your ¼ cup of chopped onions, and your tablespoon of lime juice.

4. Stir everything together well, and cook for another 5 minutes.

5. Serve when ready.

Nutritional Information:

Calories: 198

Total Fat: 7 g

Saturated Fat: 4g

Cholesterol: 35 mg

Total Carbs: 20 g

Sugar: 1 g

Fiber: 2 g

Sodium: 233 mg

Protein: 5 g

Ketogenic Deviled Eggs

They say that the devil is in the details, but he's also apparently in these deviled eggs!

Prep Time: 4 min and 30 seconds

Passive Time: 0 min

Cook Time: 0 min

Total: 4 min and 30 seconds

Serves: 5-6

Ingredients:

- 11 eggs
- ½ cup of mayonnaise
- 1 tsp of mustard
- ½ tsp of sea salt
- ¼ cup of crabmeat
- 1 tsp cayenne pepper

Directions:

1. Take a large saucepan and place it onto a burner set for high heat.

2. Now add your 3 cups of water and deposit your eggs inside the pan, and cook for about 10 minutes.

3. After 10 minutes have passed, peel the shells off the boiled eggs, and cut them in half.

4. Now take the egg yolks out, and place them in a blender, and blend them together for about 30 seconds.

5. Transfer the blended yolks to a small bowl and add your ½ cup of mayonnaise, tsp of mustard, and your ½ tsp of sea salt, stirring all of these ingredients together well.

6. Now fill each of your halved egg whites with the yolk mixture.

7. Evenly distribute your ¼ cup of crabmeat on each of the filled eggs, and serve.

Nutritional Information:

Calories: 380

Total Fat: 35 g

Saturated Fat: 1g

Cholesterol: 45 mg

Total Carbs: 1 g

Sugar: 2 g

Fiber: 0.5 g

Sodium: 239 mg

Protein: 15 g

Side of Mustard Greens

Have a Side of Mustard Greens!

Prep Time: 5 min

Passive Time: 0 min

Cook Time: 25 min

Total: 30 min

Serves: 2-3

Ingredients:

- 2 tablespoons of olive oil

- 1 cup of water

- 5 scallions, diced

- 1 tablespoon of chopped garlic

- 2 tablespoons of chicken broth

- 2 pounds of mustard greens

- 1 tablespoon of lime juice

- ½ tsp of sea salt

Directions:

1. Place a pot on a burner set for medium heat, and add your cup of water, your 2 tablespoons of olive oil, your 5 scallions, diced, your tablespoon of chopped garlic, your 2 tablespoons of chicken broth, your 2 pounds of mustard greens, your tablespoon of lime juice, and your ½ tsp of sea salt.

2. Stir and cook these ingredients for about 25 minutes.

Nutritional Information:

Calories: 128

Total Fat: 5 g

Saturated Fat: 2g

Cholesterol: 8 mg

Total Carbs: 7 g

Sugar: 1 g

Fiber: 4 g

Sodium: 157 mg

Protein: 5 g

Side of Bacon and Sugar Snap Peas

With generous portions of sugar and bacon—
these peas really are a snap!

Prep Time: 4 min

Passive Time: 0 min

Cook Time: 5 min

Total: 9 min

Serves: 1-2

Ingredients:

- 3 cups of sugar snap peas
- 1 tablespoon of lemon juice
- 3 tablespoons of bacon fat
- 1 tablespoon of chopped garlic
- 1 tsp of red pepper flakes

Directions:

1. Add your 3 tablespoons of bacon fat to a medium sized frying pan, and place the pan onto a burner set for medium-high heat.

2. Next, add your tablespoon of chopped garlic, followed by your 3 cups of sugar snap peas, and your tablespoon of lemon juice.

3. Stir and cook together for about 5 minutes.

4. Turn off your burner and season with your tsp of red pepper flakes

5. Serve whenever you are ready to do so.

Nutritional Information:

Calories: 147

Total Fat: 12 g

Saturated Fat: 2 g

Cholesterol: 23 mg

Total Carbs: 12 g

Sugar: 5 g

Fiber: 3 g

Sodium: 89 mg

Protein: 10 g

Side of Cheesy Spinach

This is a cheesy spinach blend for all seasons!

Prep Time: 3 min

Passive Time: 0 min

Cook Time: 5 min

Total: 8 min

Serves: 1-2

Ingredients:

- 5 cups of spinach
- 1 cup of shredded cheddar cheese
- 3 tablespoons of Mrs. Dash
- ½ tsp of salt
- ½ tsp of pepper
- 3 tablespoons of butter

Directions:

1. Take out a medium sized frying pan and add your 3 tablespoons of butter, followed by your 5 cups of spinach your 3 tablespoons of Mrs. Dash, your ½ tsp of salt, and your ½ tsp of pepper.

2. Set the burner to medium-high heat, and stir ingredients around in the butter as they cook for 5 minutes.

3. Finally, top the ingredients with your cup of shredded cheddar cheese, and serve!

Nutritional Information:

Calories: 352

Total Fat: 24 g

Saturated Fat: 4g

Cholesterol: 94 mg

Total Carbs: 2 g

Sugar: 3 g

Fiber: 2 g

Sodium: 234 mg

Protein: 12 g

Ketogenic Chili

Have some chili with a little bit of style!

Prep Time: 5 min

Passive Time: 0 min

Cook Time: 10 min

Total: 15 min

Serves: 1-2

Ingredients:

- 2 pounds of ground meat
- 1 cup of chopped onion
- ½ cup of chopped green bell pepper
- 1 cup of beef broth
- ¼ cup of tomato paste
- 2 tablespoons of soy sauce
- 2 tablespoons of olive oil
- 2 tablespoons of chili powder
- 1 tsp of cumin

- 2 tsp of red boat fish sauce

- 1 tablespoon of chopped garlic

- 1 tsp of paprika

- 1 tsp of oregano

- 1 tsp of cayenne pepper

- 1 tsp of Worcestershire

Directions:

1. Place a medium sized frying pan onto a burner set for high heat and add your 2 pounds of ground meat.

2. Next add your cup of chopped onion, your ½ cup of chopped green bell pepper, your cup of beef broth, your ¼ cup of tomato paste, your 2 tablespoons of soy sauce, your 2 tablespoons of olive oil, your 2 tablespoons of chili powder, your tsp of cumin, your 2 tsp of red boat fish sauce, your tablespoon of chopped garlic, your tsp of paprika, your tsp of

oregano, your tsp of cayenne pepper, and your tsp of Worcestershire.

3. Stir all of these ingredients together well as they cook over the course of the next 10 minutes.

4. Serve up your Ketogenic Chili whenever you are ready to do so.

Nutritional Information:

Calories: 321

Total Fat: 23 g

Saturated Fat: 9 g

Cholesterol: 82 mg

Total Carbs: 6 g

Sugar: 3 g

Fiber: 2 g

Sodium: 337 mg

Protein: 29 g

Red Pepper Salad

With a bit of red pepper spice over scrumptious spinach leaves! If you need a good salad--- you've just got try Red Pepper salad.

Prep Time: 3 min

Passive Time: 0 min

Cook Time: 0 min

Total: 3 min

Serves: 1-2

Ingredients:

- 3 cups of spinach
- 2 tablespoons of ranch dressing
- 1 tablespoon of parmesan cheese
- ½ tsp of red pepper flakes

Directions:

1. First, add your 3 cups of spinach to a medium sized mixing bowl, followed by your 2 tablespoons of ranch dressing.

2. Finally, top with your tablespoon of parmesan cheese, and your ½ tsp of red pepper flakes, and this Red Pepper Salad is ready to serve!

Nutritional Information:

Calories: 201

Total Fat: 17 g

Saturated Fat: 4g

Cholesterol: 15 mg

Total Carbs: 6 g

Sugar: 2 g

Fiber: 2 g

Sodium: 278 mg

Protein: 5 g

Chapter 5: Ketogenic Drinks and Dessert

At the end of yet another successful ketogenic day, you should reward yourself. Here in this chapter we present to you a listing of some of the best Ketogenic drinks and desserts you could ever hope to find. Be sure to make room in your meal plan for at least one of these great recipes.

Chocolate Puffins

Let me introduce to you some of the best ketogenic puffy muffins out there—Chocolate Puffins! Making full use of its unique ingredients, this dish delivers!

Prep Time: 7 min

Passive Time: 0 min

Cook Time: 25 min

Total: 32 min

Serves: 4-5

Ingredients:

- 2 tsp cream of tartar
- 1 tsp of sea salt
- 12 eggs
- ½ cup of Confectioners Swerve
- 1 tsp of chocolate extract
- 3 tablespoons of cocoa powder

Directions:

1. Set your oven for 375 degrees.
2. Add your 3 tablespoons of cocoa powder, your tsp of chocolate extract, and your ½ cup of Confectioners Swerve

to a small bowl and stir the ingredients together.

3. Now get out a separate, large-sized mixing bowl and add your 12 eggs, your tsp of sea salt, and your 1 tsp cream of tartar and stir the ingredients together.

4. Dump your cocoa powder mixture into the larger bowl and stir everything again, one more time.

5. Pour the mixture into the cups of a greased muffin tin and place into the oven.

6. Set the oven temperature for 350 degrees and cook the muffins for about 25 minutes, or until golden brown on top.

Nutritional Information:

Calories: 208

Total Fat: 15 g

Saturated Fat: 1g

Cholesterol: 23 mg

Total Carbs: 3 g

Sugar: 5 g

Fiber: 1 g

Sodium: 235 mg

Protein: 16 g

Creamy Strawberry Popsicles

These creamy popsicles go down smooth and satisfying!

Prep Time: 10 min

Passive Time: 1 hour and 30 min

Cook Time: 0 min

Total: 1 hour and 40 min

Serves: 4

Ingredients:

- 4 ounces of cream cheese

- ¼ cup of almond milk

- 4 tablespoons of Confectioners Swerve

- 1 tsp of strawberry extract

Directions:

1. Deposit your 4 ounces of cream cheese, your ¼ cup of almond milk, your 4

tablespoons of Confectioners Swerve, and your tsp of strawberry extract into a medium sized mixing bowl and stir the ingredients together well.

2. Next, pour the mixture into "popsicle molds" you should be able to make at least 4 popsicles.

3. Freeze for about 1 hour and 30 minutes.

4. Once frozen, take out of the fridge and enjoy!

Nutritional Information:

Calories: 103

Total Fat: 10 g

Saturated Fat: 1g

Cholesterol: 67 mg

Total Carbs: 1 g

Sugar: 4 g

Fiber: 0.5 g

Sodium: 55 mg

Protein: 2 g

Strawberry Milkshake

If you are on a real strawberry kick—liven things up with a Strawberry Milkshake! And thanks to ketogenic, this rendition won't wreck your diet!

Prep Time: 3 min and 30 seconds
Passive Time: 0 min
Cook Time: 0 min
Total: 3 min and 30 seconds

Serves: 4

Ingredients:

- 8 ounces of cream cheese
- 1 cup of almond milk
- ¼ cup of Confectioners Swerve sweetener
- 1 tsp of vanilla extract
- 1 tsp of strawberry extract

- 1 cup of crushed ice

- 1 tsp of Aloe Vera juice

Directions:

1. Deposit your 8 ounces of cream cheese, your cup of almond milk, your ¼ cup of Confectioners Swerve, your tsp of vanilla extract, your tsp of strawberry extract, your cup of crushed ice, and your tsp of Aloe Vera juice.

2. Press the blend button, and blend for about 1 minute and 30 seconds.

3. Pour into glasses and serve.

Nutritional Information:

Calories: 200

Total Fat: 19 g

Saturated Fat: 3g

Cholesterol: 92 mg

Total Carbs: 9 g

Sugar: 5 g

Fiber: 0.5 g

Sodium: 29 mg

Protein: 4 g

Ketogenic Chocolate Pots De Crème

Is it ice cream? Is it a shake? Cocoa? Oh no, it's none of those—it's simply Ketogenic Chocolate Pots De Crème!

Prep Time: 7 min
Passive Time: 45 min
Cook Time: 0 min
Total: 52 min

Serves: 2

Ingredients:

- 2 cups of coconut milk
- 3 tablespoons of Confectioners Swerve
- 3 tablespoons of cocoa powder
- 1 tablespoon of gelatin
- 1 tsp of vanilla extract
- ½ tsp of almond extract
- ½ tsp of sea salt

Directions:

1. Add about 1 cup of your coconut milk to a medium sized mixing bowl, followed by your tablespoon of gelatin.

2. Briefly stir and set the mixture to the side.

3. Next, place a medium sized saucepan onto a burner set for high heat and add your remaining cup of coconut milk to the pan.

4. Now add your 3 tablespoons of cocoa powder, your Confectioners Swerve, your tsp of almond extract, and your tsp of sea salt to the pan, stirring everything together well.

5. Turn off your burner and pour the mixture into 2 separate serving cups, and place them inside your refrigerator.

6. Let them sit inside your fridge to chill for about 45 minutes before serving.

Nutritional Information:

Calories: 210

Total Fat: 18 g

Saturated Fat: 9g

Cholesterol: 53 mg

Total Carbs: 8 g

Sugar: 7 g

Fiber: 2 g

Sodium: 27 mg

Protein: 10 g

Bullet Proof Ketogenic Coffee

This great coffee keeps you up without the carbs! Atjust 1 carb per serving—this coffee really is bullet proof!

Prep Time: 3 min

Passive Time: 15seconds

Cook Time: 1 min

Total: 4 min and 15 seconds

Serves: 1

Ingredients:

- 1 cup of coffee
- 1 tablespoon of unsalted butter
- 1 tablespoon of coconut oil
- 1 tablespoon of heavy cream

Directions:

1. Start off by brewing yourself a cup of coffee, should take around 1 minute.

2. Next, add your tablespoon of unsalted butter to the coffee, allowing it to settle into the cup of about 15 seconds.

3. Now add your tablespoon of coconut oil, followed by your tablespoon of heavy cream.

4. Stir all of these ingredients together well and you have yourself a cup of Bullet Proof Ketogenic Coffee!

Nutritional Information:

Calories: 145

Total Fat: 8 g

Saturated Fat: 1 g

Cholesterol: 31 mg

Total Carbs: 1 g

Sugar: 4 g

Fiber: 2 g

Sodium: 20 mg

Protein: 1 g

Spicy Mug Coffee Cake

If you would like to have some cake with your coffee in the morning, just get a load of this Spicy Mug Coffee Cake! You'll be the envy of the break room with this one!

Prep Time: 3 min
Passive Time: 0 min
Cook Time: 55seconds
Total: 3 min and 55 seconds

Serves: 1

Ingredients:

- 1 egg
- 2 tablespoons of butter
- 4 tablespoons of almond flour
- 1 tablespoon of NOW Erythritol
- 5 drops of liquid stevia
- ½ tsp of baking powder

- ½ tsp of cinnamon

- ½ tsp of ginger

- ½ tsp of clove

- ½ tsp of cardamom

- ½ tsp of vanilla extract

Directions:

1. Deposit your egg, followed by your 2 tablespoons of butter, your 4 tablespoons of almond flour, your tablespoon of NOW Erythritol, your 5 drops of liquid stevia, your ½ tsp of baking powder, your ½ tsp of baking powder, your ½ tsp of ginger, your ½ tsp of clove, your ½ tsp of cardamom, and your ½ tsp of vanilla extract.

2. Stir everything together well before placing the mug into the microwave, and cooking it for 55 seconds.

3. Once cooked, take the mug out (careful its hot) and turn it upside down over a bowl or plate, allowing the cooked cake to slide right out.

4. Sprinkle your ½ tsp of cinnamon on top for flavor, and serve!

Nutritional Information:

Calories: 155

Total Fat: 5 g

Saturated Fat: 1g

Cholesterol: 4 mg

Total Carbs: 25 g

Sugar: 5 g

Fiber: 1.5 g

Sodium: 178 mg

Protein: 3 g

Ketogenic-Doodle Cookies

If you like snicker doodle cookies—then you are absolutely going to love Ketogenic-Doodle Cookies! It tastes just like the original, but without the carbs!

Prep Time: 7 min
Passive Time: 0 min
Cook Time: 10 min
Total: 17 min

Serves: 6-7

Ingredients:

- 2 cups of almond flour
- ¼ cup of coconut oil
- 1 tablespoon of maple syrup
- 1 tablespoon of vanilla
- 1 tsp of baking powder
- 2 tablespoons of cinnamon

- ¼ tsp of salt

- 1 tsp of stevia

Directions:

1. Set your oven's temperature to 385 degrees.

2. Take out a medium sized mixing bowl and add your 2 cups of almond flour, your tsp of baking soda, and your ¼ tsp of salt, mixing them together well.

3. Now get out an additional bowl and add your ¼ cup of coconut oil, your tablespoon of maple syrup, your tsp of stevia, and your tablespoon of vanilla

4. Stir these together before pouring the mixture out into your mixing bowl of flour ingredients.

5. Now add your 2 tablespoons of cinnamon to the mix, and with your (clean) hands, shape the ingredients into small balls of dough.

6. Place these balls of dough onto a greased cooking sheet, before taking a roller pin to them to make them flat.

7. Now put the sheet into the oven and cook the dough for about 10 minutes.

8. Once cooked, take out of the oven and serve immediately!

Nutritional Information:

Calories: 137

Total Fat: 12 g

Saturated Fat: 2g

Cholesterol: 22 mg

Total Carbs: 14 g

Sugar: 4 g

Fiber: 1 g

Sodium: 50 mg

Protein: 7 g

Lemon Cake Moon Pies

Lemon Cake Moon Pies? Well this one certainly brings back some good memories! If you used to enjoy those moon pie treats of yesteryear, then you should give this fantastic little recipe a try!

Prep Time: 8 min
Passive Time: 0 min
Cook Time: 10 min
Total: 18 min

Serves: 4-5

Ingredients:

- ¼ cup of almond flour
- ¼ cup of coconut flour
- ¼ cup of butter
- 3 eggs
- ¼ cup of Erythritol

- 1 tablespoon of lemon juice

- 1 tablespoon of coconut milk

- 1 tsp of cinnamon

- ½ tsp of almond extract

- ½ tsp of vanilla extract

- ½ tsp of baking soda

- ½ tsp of apple cider vinegar

- ¼ tsp of liquid stevia

- ¼ tsp of salt

- 4 ounces of cream cheese

- 4 tablespoons of butter

- 2 tablespoons of heavy cream

- 1 tablespoon of red food coloring

Directions:

1. Set your oven for 330 degrees.

2. While your oven is warming up, add your ¼ cup of coconut flour, your ¼ cup of almond flour, your ¼ tsp of salt, your

½ tsp of baking soda, and your 1 tsp of cinnamon.

3. Next, add your 3 eggs, your ¼ cup of Erythritol, your ½ tsp of vanilla extract, your ½ tsp of almond extract, your tablespoon of lemon juice, your tablespoon of coconut milk, your ½ tsp of apple cider vinegar, your ¼ tsp of stevia, and your tablespoon of red food coloring, mixing these ingredients together as well, stirring everything until it becomes one fine batter.

4. Now take out a greased muffin tin and evenly distribute the batter between the greased cups of the tin.

5. Place muffin tin into the oven and cook for about 10 minutes.

6. Once cooked take the muffins out of the cups, and cut each one of them in half, horizontally across, and set them to the side for a moment.

7. Next, take out another mixing bowl and add your 4 ounces of cream cheese, your 4 tablespoons of butter, and your 2 tablespoons of heavy cream.

8. Stir these ingredients together well and evenly fill each of your sliced muffins with this mixture.

9. Your Lemon Cake Moon Pies are complete!

Nutritional Information:

Calories: 180

Total Fat: 17 g

Saturated Fat: 2g

Cholesterol: 32 mg

Total Carbs: 3 g

Sugar: 4 g

Fiber: 1 g

Sodium: 49 mg

Protein: 3 g

Conclusion: Ketogenic and Loving It!

Besides the obvious benefit of getting your body to burn fat, and successfully lose weight—the reason why the ketogenic diet is so well received, is because it uses a completely open template in its implementation. Ketogenic does not base itself on a rigid set of rules that every single dieter must follow. The main goal of the diet is to get your body into a metabolic state of ketosis, so it can burn fat. Exactly how you reach this goal is completely up to you.

As this book has demonstrated there are several ways in which you can arrange your meal plans and ingredients in order to reach ketosis. And as such, this book provides a diverse batch of recipes, allowing you to pick and choose which would work best for your schedule, your energy needs, and your own personal taste. This book simply gives you the tools you need to make ketogenic a reality for yourself, and how you use those tools is entirely up to you. Whether you are committing yourself for a week, month, year, or a lifetime, it's up to you how you maintain your ketogenic diet.

We all have preferences, and individualized tastes, and this book has taken all of that into account. So, you don't have to worry too much about the exact details of how you engage in your diet, you can chart your own course. Really, all you need to do, all you need to understand, and all you need to know, is that this cookbook you hold in your hand—is simply ketogenic! Thank you for reading!